FUCK CANCER COLORING BOOK FOR ADULTS

GOOD VIBES COLORING BOOK FOR CANCER SURVIVORS AND PATIENTS

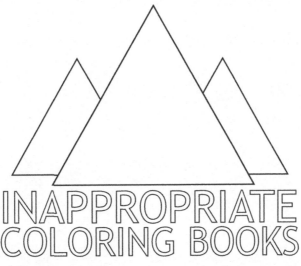

INAPPROPRIATE
COLORING BOOKS

ISBN: 9781694420763
Imprint: Independently published

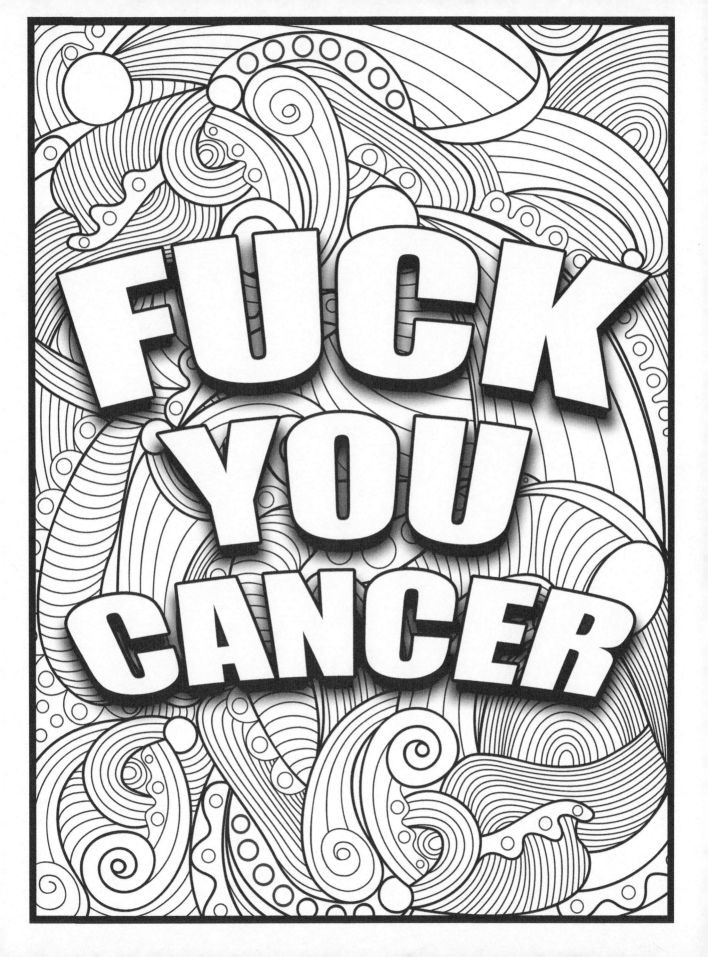

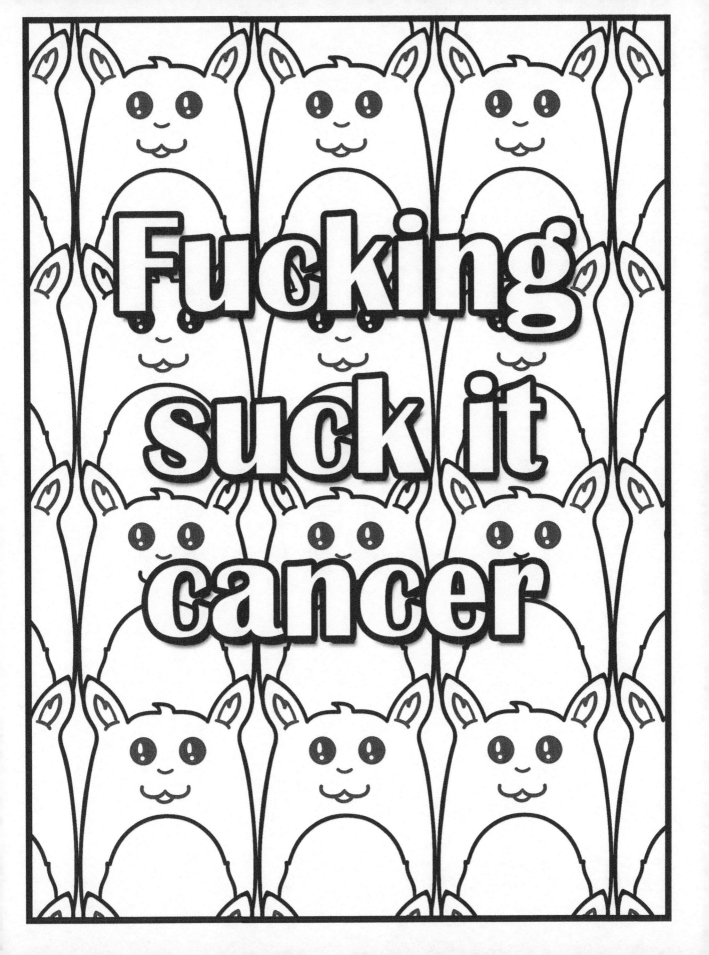

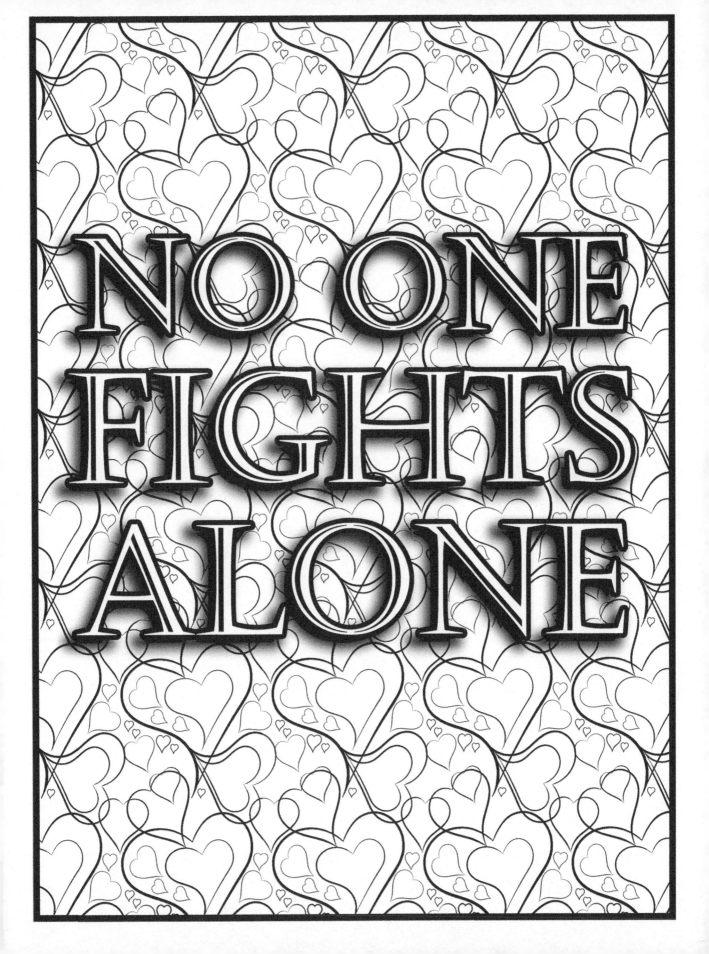

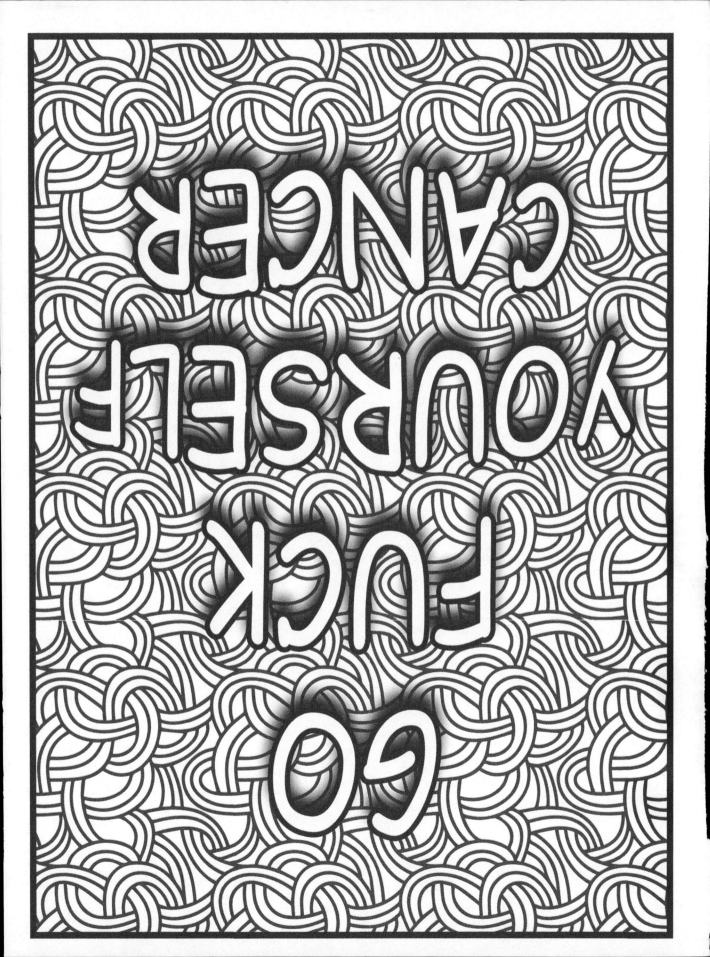

The C in Cancer stands for CUNT

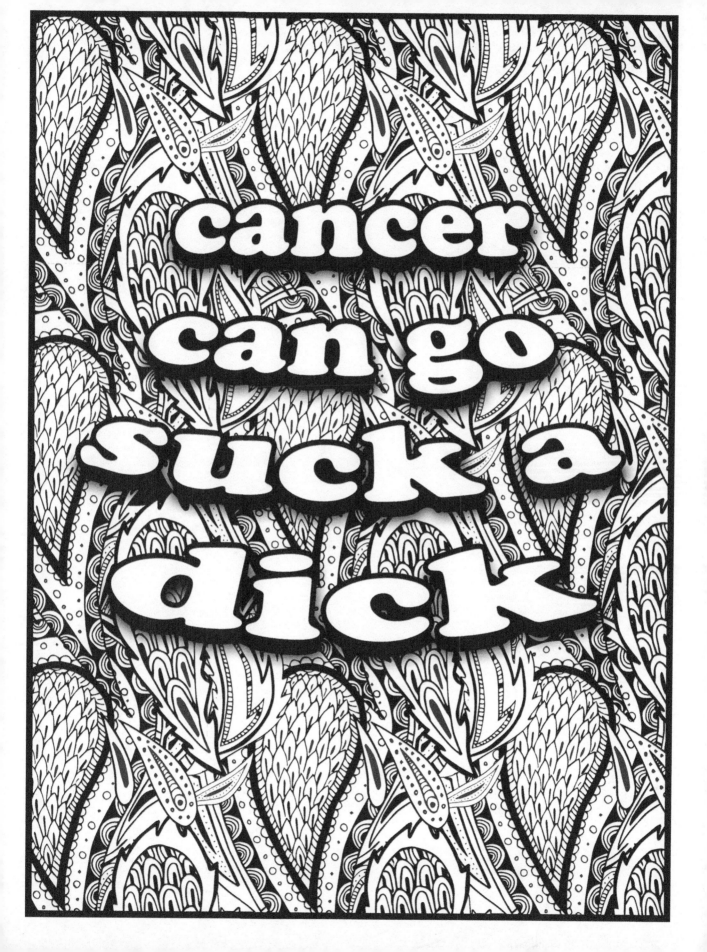

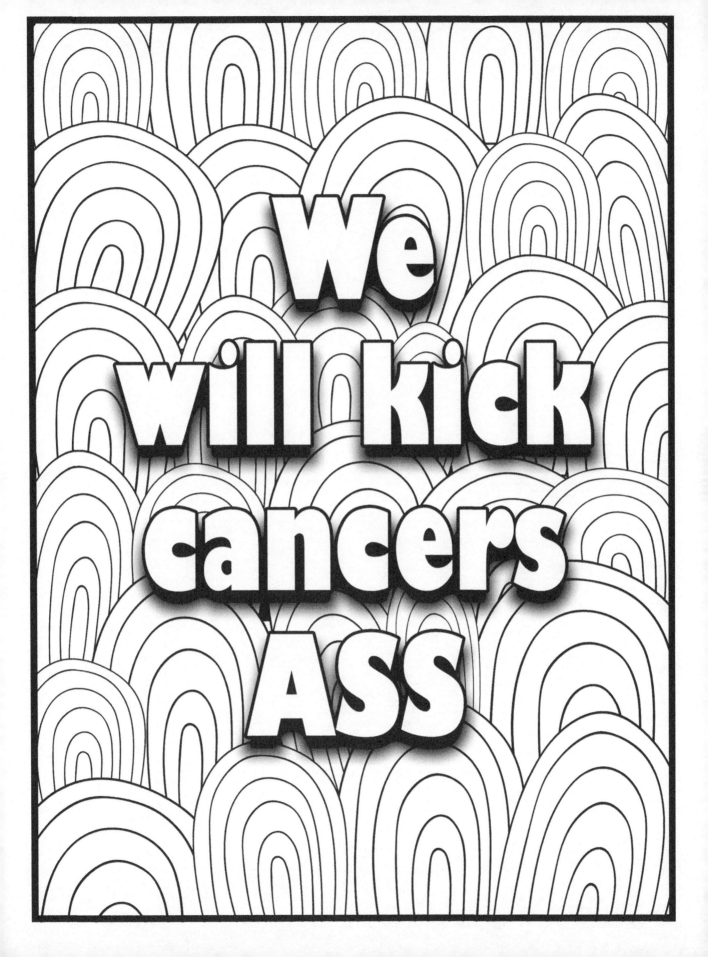

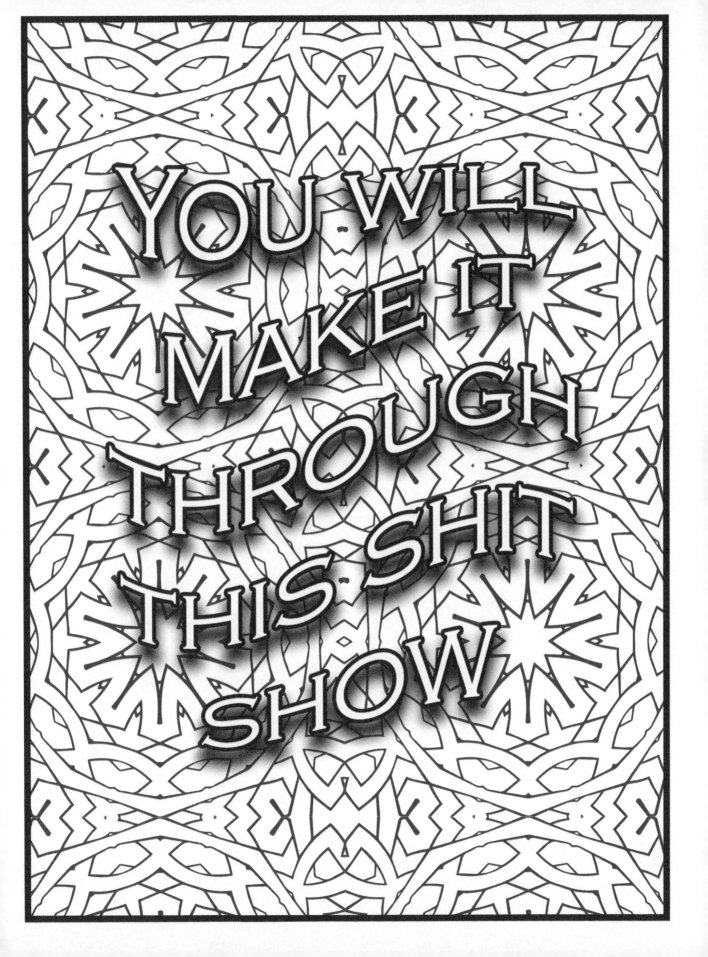

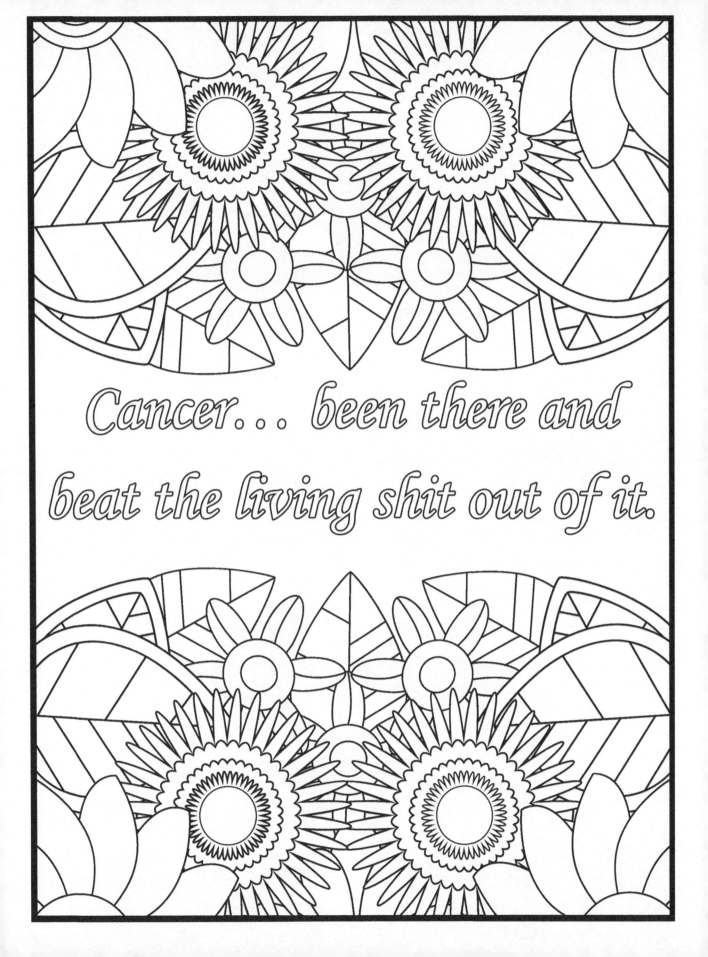

Cancer... been there and beat the living shit out of it.

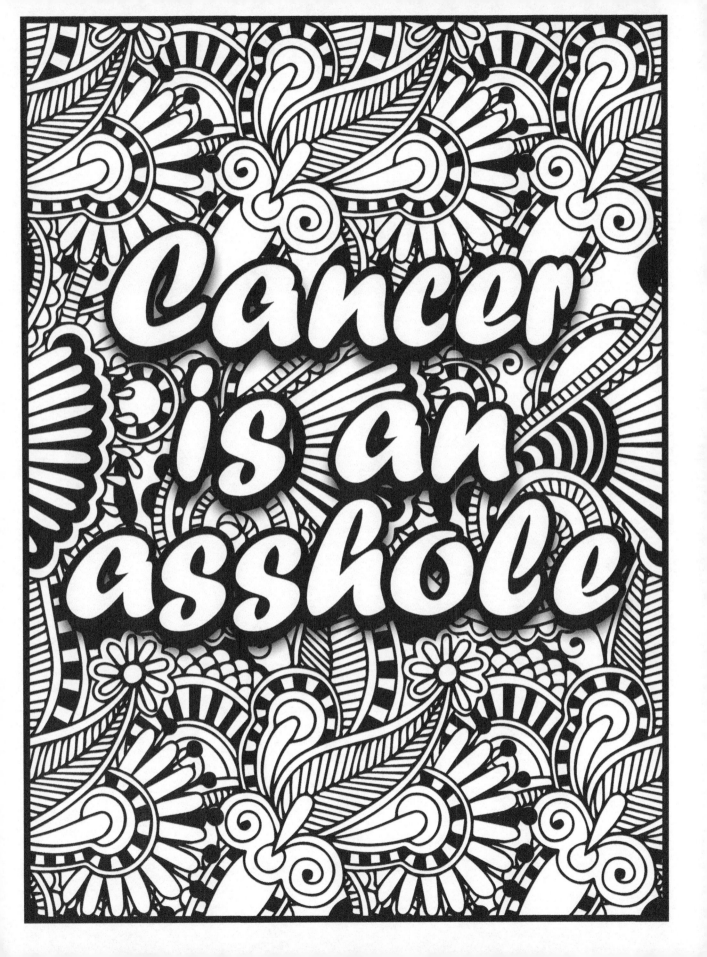

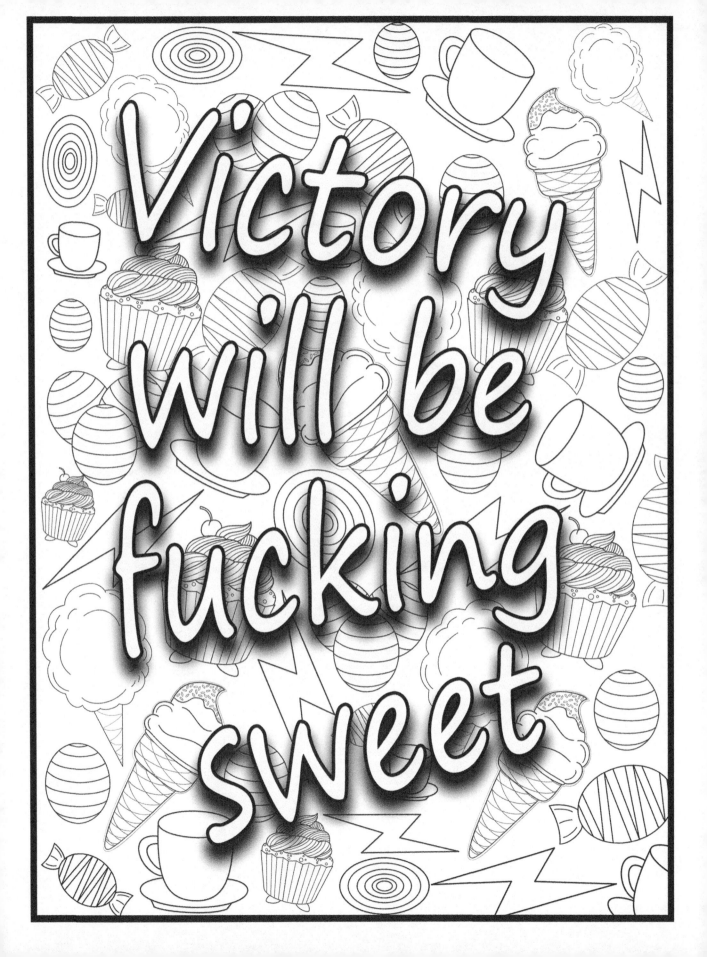

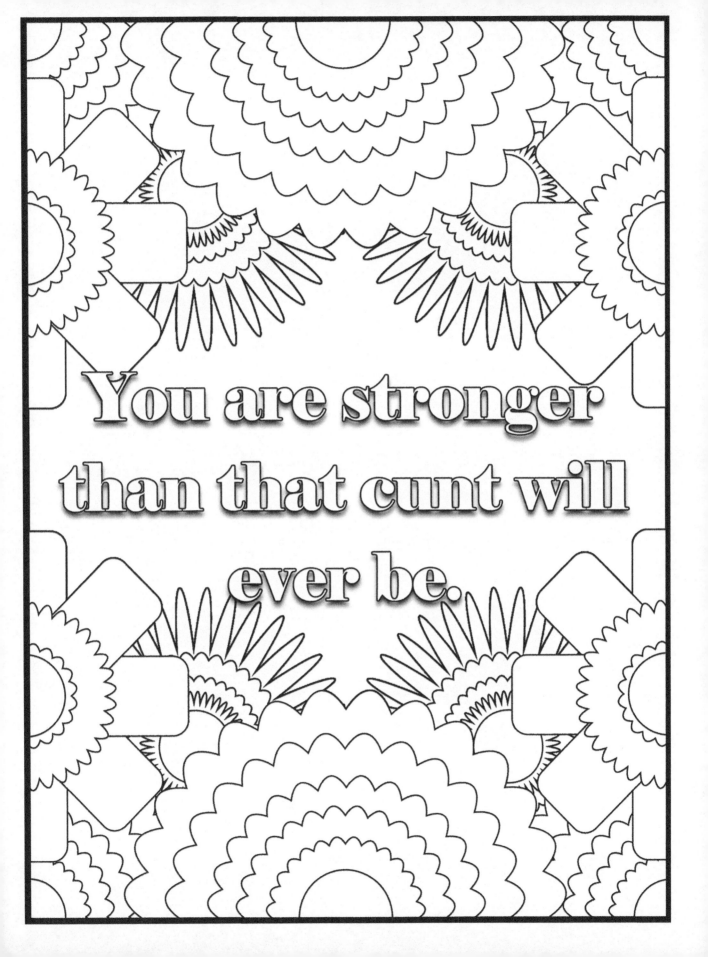

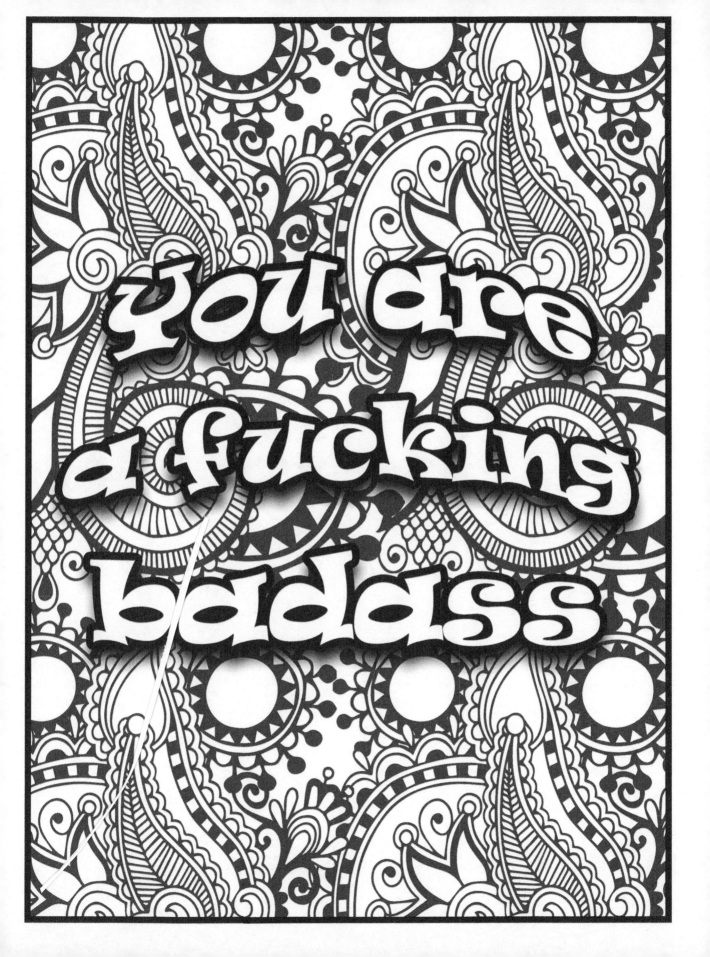

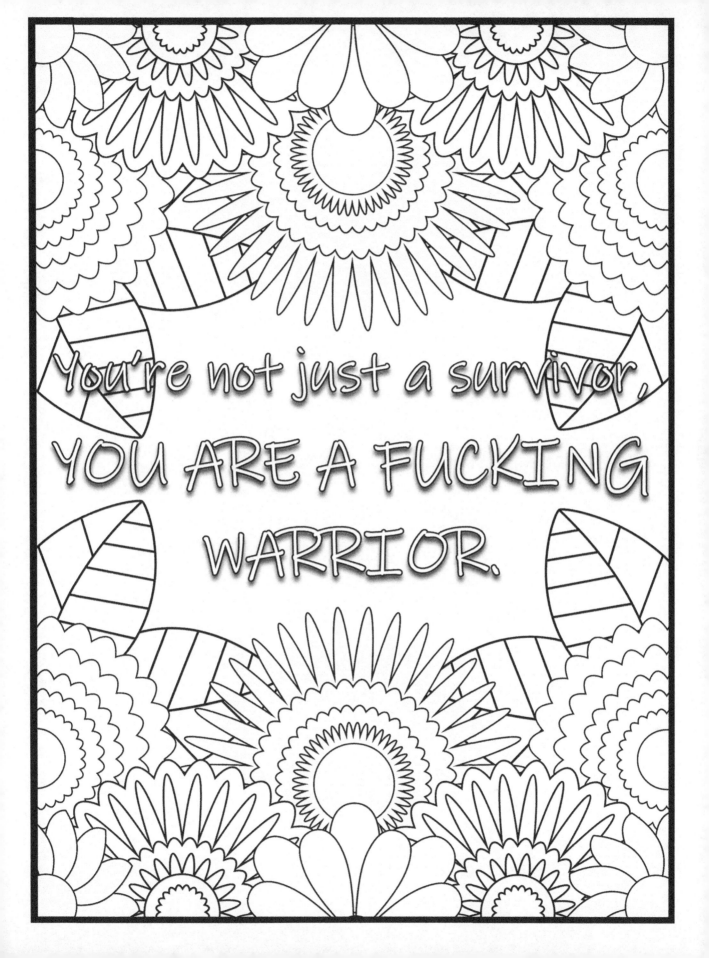

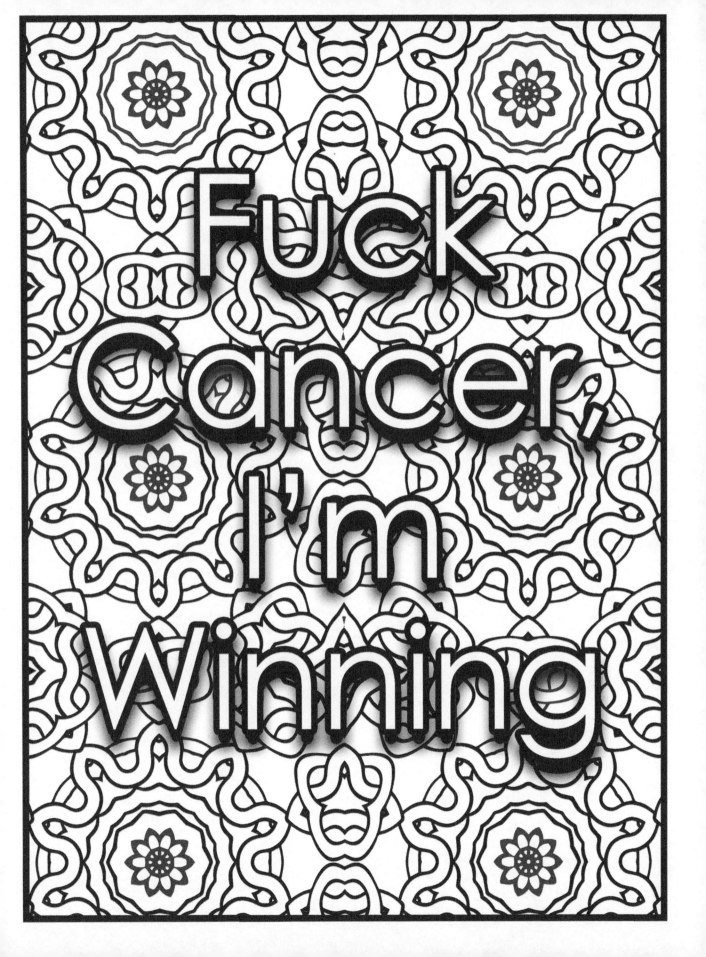

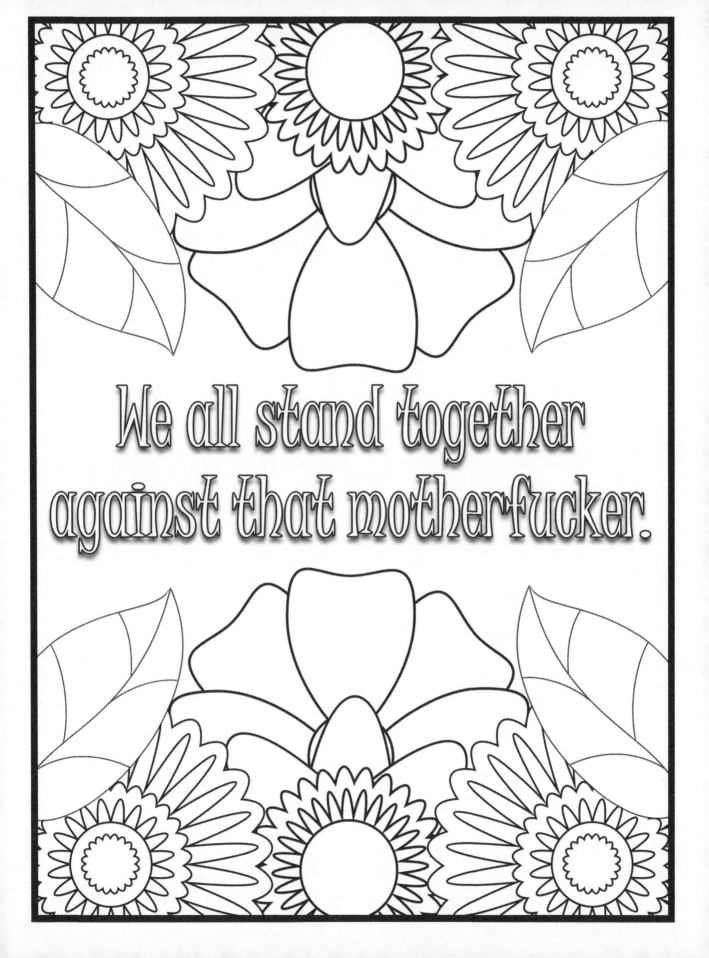

We all stand together against that motherfucker.

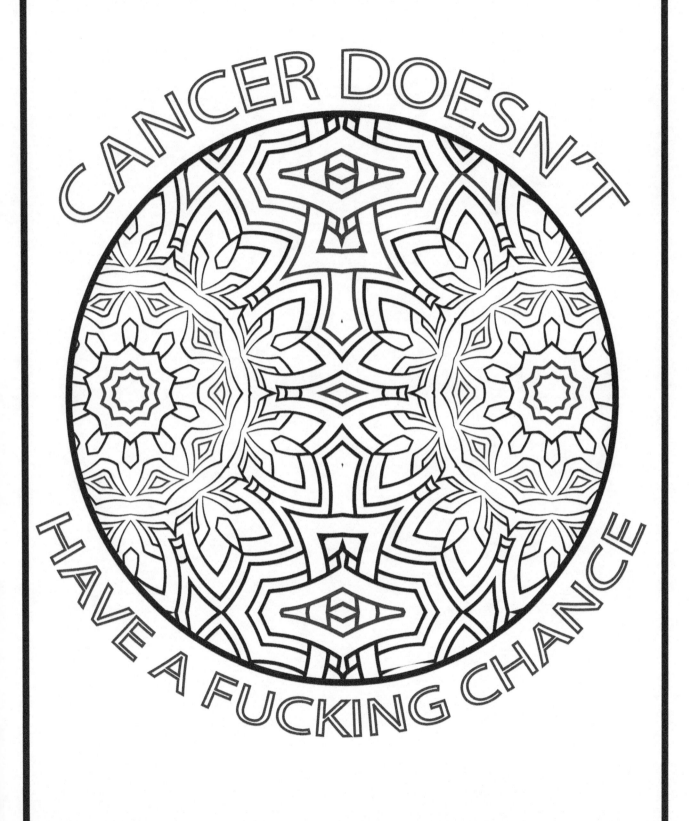

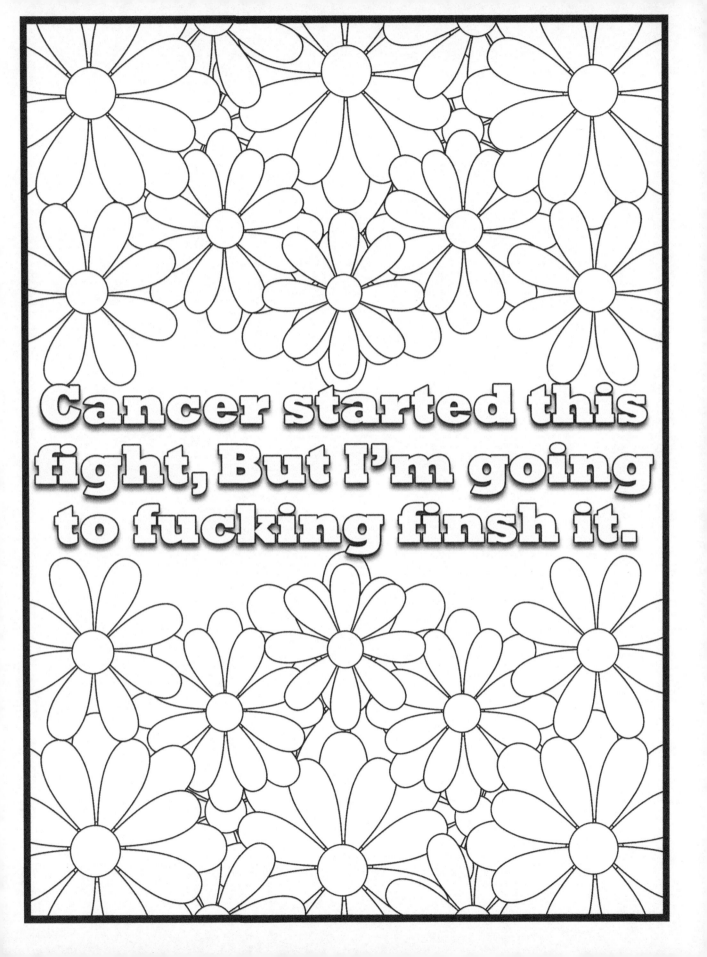

Fight like a fucking boss

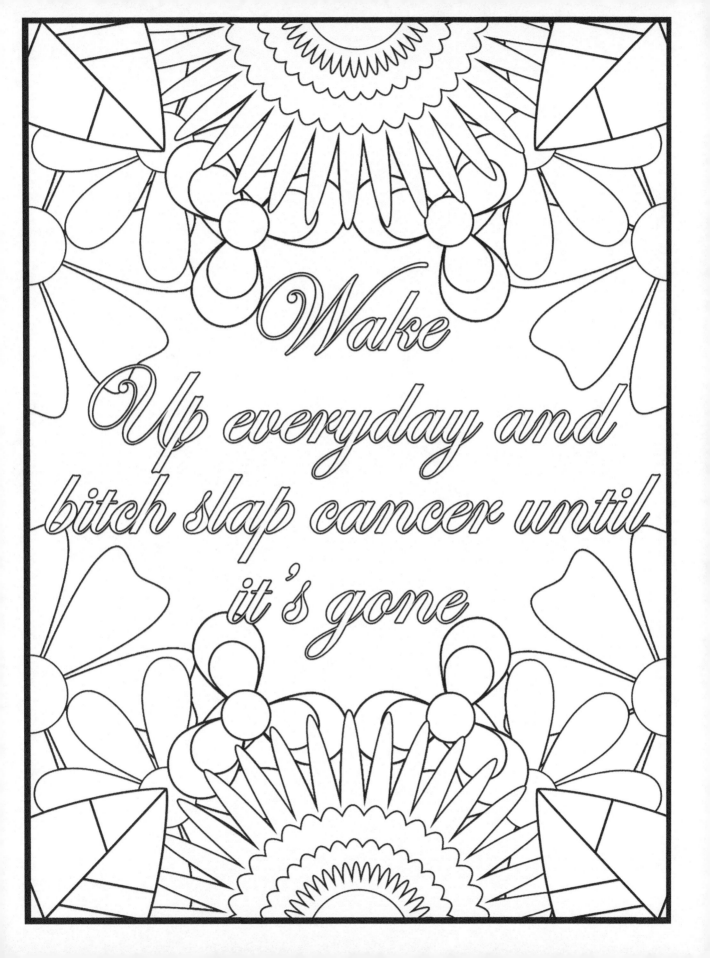

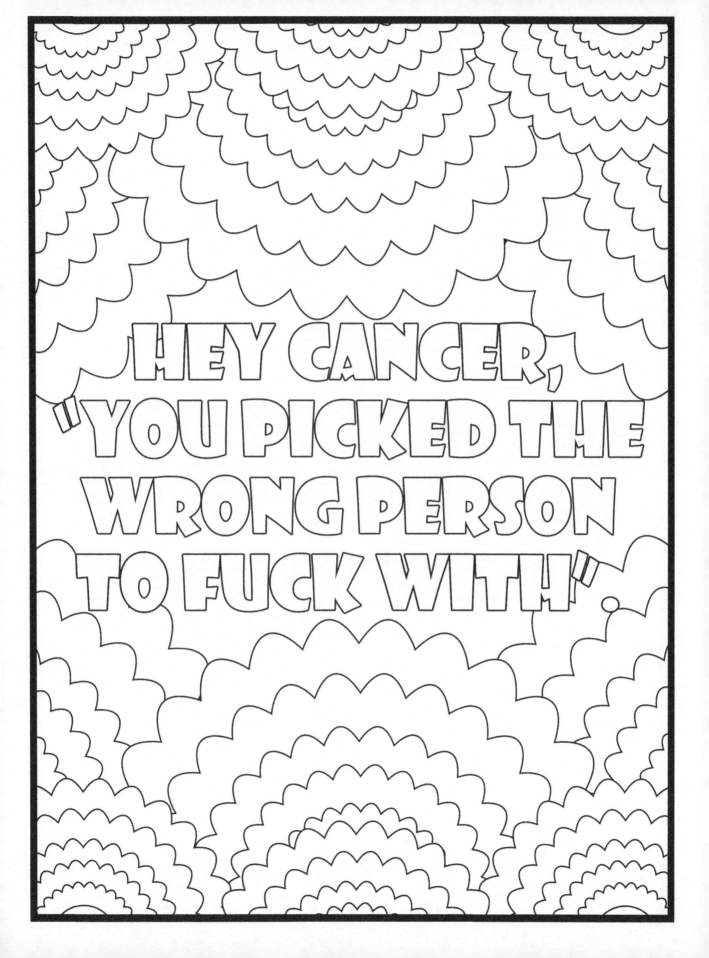

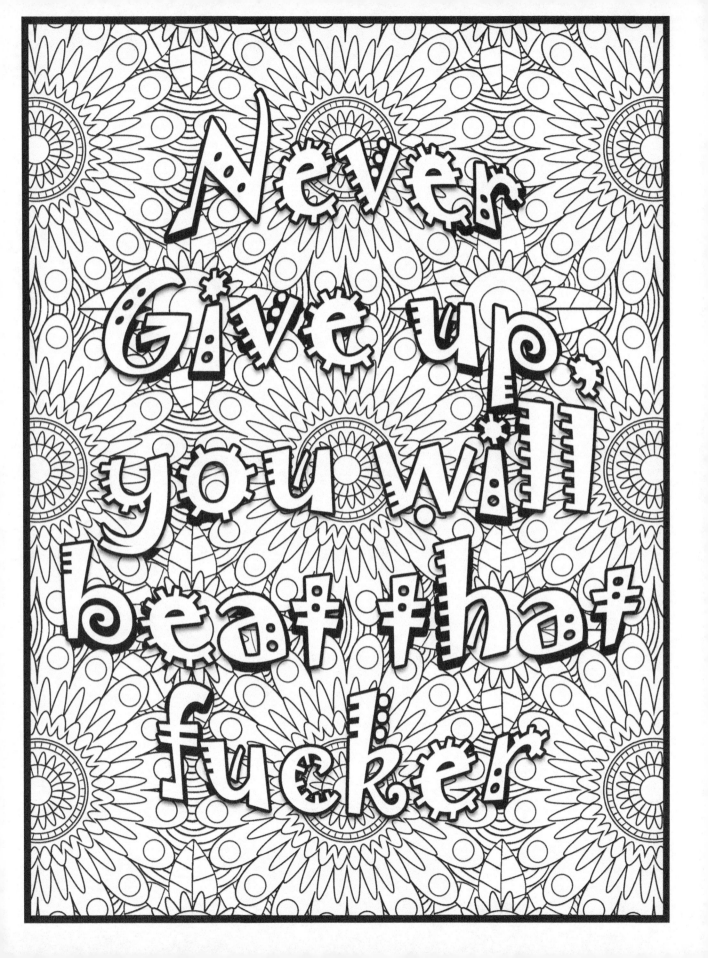

Cancer touched my boobs so I kicked its ass

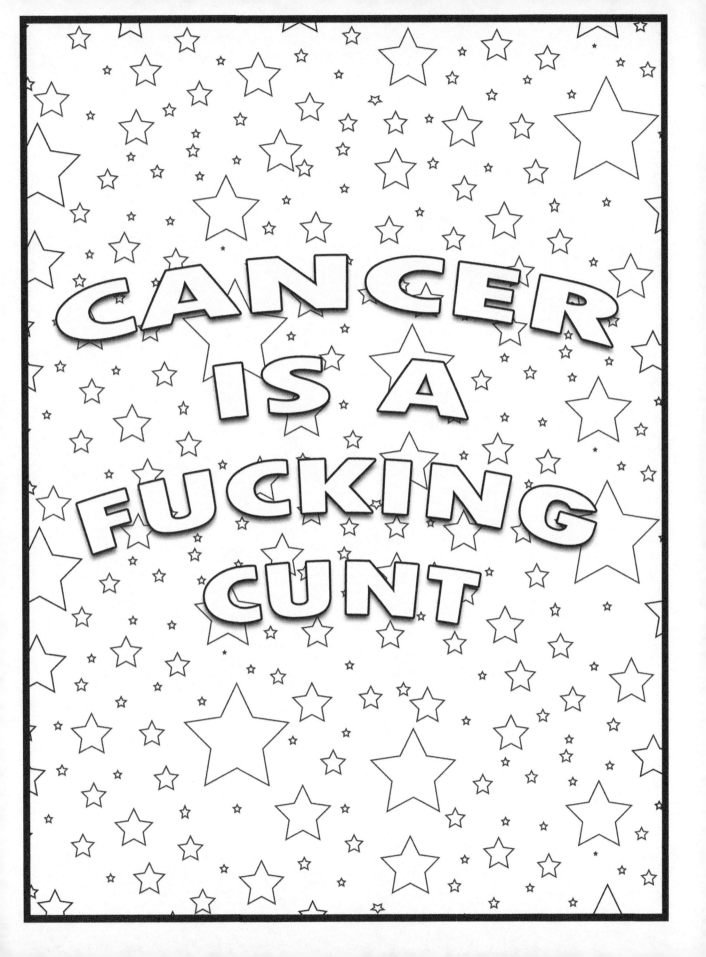

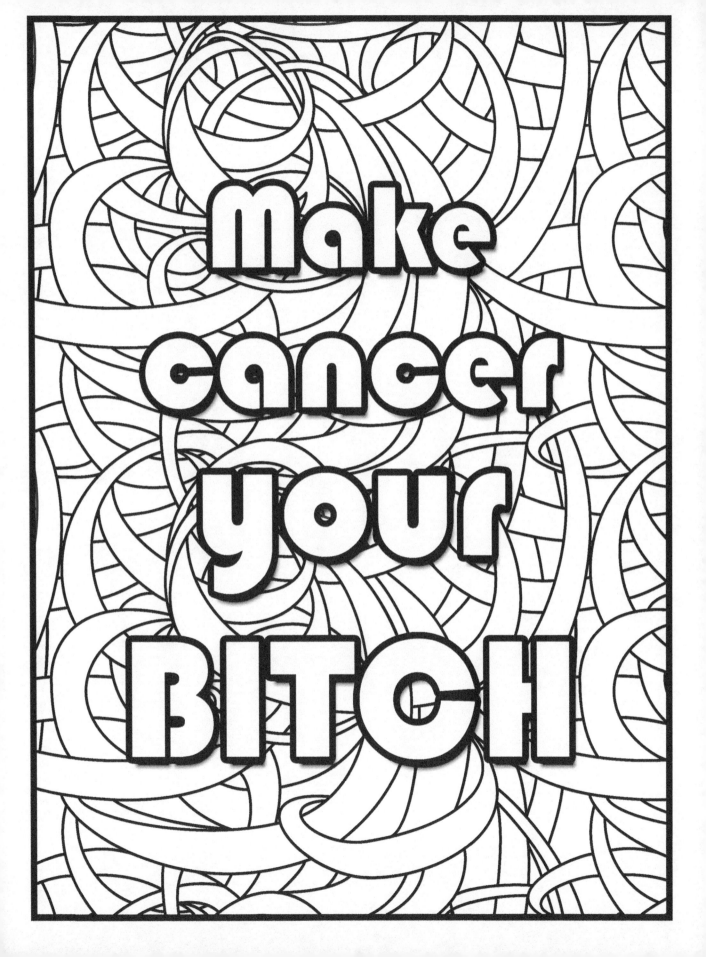

COLOR TEST PAGE

COLOR TEST PAGE

Made in the USA
Monee, IL
25 November 2022

18529418R00033